A Physician-Patient Guidebook for a Weight Control Program

A Physician-Patient Guidebook for a Weight Control Program

Dr Charles J. Neilson MD

Foreward

Hello, I am Dr Charles J. Neilson MD, a former Family Physician for 21 years in Houston, Texas. During those years, I developed an approach to weight reduction which I found highly successful with my private practice patients. I found out early in my practice that I was ill-prepared to help obese patients lose weight effectively. My Family Practice residency training experience in the 1970's regarding weight reduction and weight control had been incomplete, if not archaic, and in 1977 I was taught the following guidelines: 1) Limit calorie restrictions to no less than 1200-1500 calories a day; 2) Never use appetite suppressants (anorectics) – "They're dangerous and addicting"; 3) Include "exercise" (without any distinction as to what kind of exercise is appropriate for weight reduction versus maintenance); 4) Include "Behavioral Modification" (without any explanation other than to suggest that I go to the library and "look it up").

Other than these guidelines, not much more was forthcoming to prepare me to help the obese patient. But I certainly remember the expert physician who was the only professor I had that actually treated obese patients. His approach was to hospitalize young obese teenage girls and keep their door locked for two weeks while cutting their daily calorie intake to around 1200 calories – and most importantly, keeping candy and junk food away. Taking all of these guidelines into my solo practice soon led to flat-out failure.

Dr Charles J. Neilson MD

Initially, my association as the Houston Police Department Boxing Team ringside physician led to an opportunity to help overweight policemen lose weight. There were limitations on an officer's weight in order to remain on the force and I was chosen by a number of obese cops to help them lose weight. So I started with very motivated patients. Unfortunately they could not stay motivated with only a two pound weight loss per week (which was the "safe" limit imposed by my training). The same problem occurred with obese housewives and other civilian patients – they would quit after 4 to 6 weeks at such a slow pace. Furthermore, they knew they could not afford to see the doctor every two weeks for close supervision over a projected year or more of tedious effort on their part.

I found that, without appetite suppressants, almost all of these patients were facing constant hunger. And with the requisite "exercise", they seemed to GAIN weight as a rule! My poor attempt to apply behavioral modification techniques did not help matters either. Overall, my training appeared to be as effective as the old approach to a prone drowning victim by pressing on the chest and then lifting their elbows up in repeated fashion. In other words, totally wrong. With complete failure regarding obese patients, I soon had to "fly by the seat of my pants". With a number of markedly obese policeman, whose jobs were jeopardized by their excessive weight, I soon developed my own approach. This surprisingly worked on nearly every obese patient I saw. Besides policemen (who are inclined to better self-discipline than average folk) over two decades, I found success with nearly every obese patient regardless of their gender or occupation.

Although late in coming, in 1992, after major adjustments in treatment, I happened to read Weintraub's (see references) medical research publication which in effect demonstrated that, essentially what I had been doing for my obese patients had been found to be very effective and was best at preventing recurrent obesity.

In 1992, in Clinical Pharmacology and Therapeutics, Dr Michael Weintraub, of the University of Rochester School of Medicine and Dentistry, described the results of his four year study that demonstrated a successful combination of calorie restraints (dieting), exercise, behavioral modification, and appetite suppressant medication. This was found to help seriously obese people lose weight and maintain that weight loss. Unfortunately, the appetite suppressant combination that he selected, phentermine and fenfluramine, ("Fen-Phen") was later tied to heart valve problems and pulmonary hypertension. Up to 30% of patients taking Fen-Phen developed heart valve damage. Although this combination of drugs was initially FDA-approved, it soon was withdrawn and many attorneys pursued doctors and drug companies.

It was fortunate on my part to have confined my use of anorectic (appetite suppressant) medication to solely phentermine in my diet plan in spite of the FDA approval of Fen-Phen. It seems that Dr Weintraub was trying to take advantage of the two different mechanisms of action of both drugs in his quest to maximize and prolong the effects of the appetite suppression part of his weight program. Having started the use of any anorectic at all (after the bias against anorectics during my earlier training years) was brave enough during my initial weight reduction program. I, thus, dodged that bullet while successfully developing my weight plan. So, I must emphasize that the hazards of Fen-Phen should not be associated with my diet plan described hereafter as I never promoted the use of Fen-Phen and always discouraged my patients from using that combination. The use of phentermine alone and without combination with phenfluramine is and has been my approach to the use of anorectics in weight reduction and continues to enjoy FDA approval.

I believe that by reading my book, not only can patients succeed in a diet program, but their own physician, who might have received the older dogmatic and ineffective approach in his or her training, might be able to better help their patients with weight control. As a testament to my self-developed approach to fast weight loss/weight control methods, I was never sued for malpractice by anyone during my two decades of seeing hundreds of weight patients. I am happy to say that the benefits of my approach are not restricted to just obese patients. I found that the program, especially the behavioral modification techniques, led to optimal motivation and success with non-obese patients as well.

Important Notice

The most important warning that I can give you is that my plan is NOT SAFE unless the patient following my weight reduction and maintenance plan is closely followed by their physician every two weeks during the weight reduction mode and periodically during weight maintenance (eg every three months). I have seen numerous patients make changes in my instructions, often from the advice of good-intentioned family and friends, and then get sick. Only by immediately calling your doctor to discuss unexpected results or untoward events should you avoid unnecessary or prolonged negative experiences that could even be dangerous. I never had a patient with an adverse event that could not be rectified quickly, however those who asked their friends for advice usually suffered unnecessarily until they finally contacted me. A fast weight program can be dangerous, even lead to death if the patient does not maintain a professional ongoing relationship with a physician who is familiar with the Weintraub studies' complete program (minus the Fen-Phen or Redux), has expertise in weight control, or has read this book.

References

Long-term weight control: the National Heart, Lung, and Blood Institute funded multimodal intervention study. Weintraub M. (medline) Clin Pharmacol Ther. 1992 May;51(5):581-5.

Dr Charles J. Neilson MD

Long-term weight control study. I (weeks 0 to 34). The enhancement of behavior modification, caloric restriction, and exercise by fenfluramine plus phentermine versus placebo. Weintraub M, et al. (medline) Clin Pharmacol Ther. 1992 May;51(5):586-94.

Long-term weight control study. II (weeks 34 to 104). An open-label study of continuous fenfluramine plus phentermine versus targeted intermittent medication as adjuncts to behavior modification, caloric restriction, and exercise. Weintraub M, et al. (medline) Clin Pharmacol Ther. 1992 May;51(5):595-601.

Long-term weight control study. III (weeks 104 to 156). An open-label study of dose adjustment of fenfluramine and phentermine. Weintraub M, et al. (medline) Clin Pharmacol Ther. 1992 May;51(5):602-7.

Long-term weight control study. IV (weeks 156 to 190). The second double-blind phase. Weintraub M, et al. (medline) Clin Pharmacol Ther. 1992 May;51(5):608-14.

Long-term weight control study. V (weeks 190 to 210). Follow-up of participants after cessation of medication. (medline) Clin Pharmacol Ther. 1992 May;51(5):615-8.

Long-term weight control study. VI. Individual participant response patterns. Weintraub M, et al. (medline) Clin Pharmacol Ther. 1992 May;51(5):619-33.

Long-term weight control study. VII (weeks 0 to 210). Serum lipid changes. Weintraub M, et al. (medline) Clin Pharmacol Ther. 1992 May;51(5):634-41.

Long-term weight control study: conclusions. Weintraub M. (medline) Clin Pharmacol Ther. 1992 May;51(5):642-6.

A double-blind clinical trial in weight control. Use of fenfluramine and phentermine alone and in combination. Weintraub M, et al. (medline) Arch Intern Med. 1984 Jun;144(6):1143-8.

Note to Physicians

If you were like me, starting out in the practice of medicine without adequate training or experience in providing effective weight control, you and your patients can obtain years of experience through reading this book. I wish I had such a guideline when I first started. Not only will you have a primer that includes all issues that are known to make a weight reduction (and ultimately, weight maintenance) program most effective, but your patients can follow the program with total understanding of the process and their responsibilities. Not only specific guidelines in providing the patient with behavioral modification training is included, but other important information is included: (1) what kind of exercise and when? (2) safe anorectic medication use (3) potassium supplementation with rapid weight loss (4) stool normalizers (5) and a multitude of analogies and patient motivation descriptions that help obese patients understand how they must think in order to succeed at weight control.

Your responsibility remains as always to evaluate each and every patient and determine their suitability for rapid weight loss versus slow weight loss. Your history taking, physical examination, and laboratory findings should dictate that certain patients are not candidates for rapid weight loss. Therefore, the very low calorie diet (see Chapter Three) will not be suitable and it will be your responsibility to limit such patients to more modest calorie restrictions (eg 1200 to 1500 calories a day.) Anorectics medicines should not be started until hypertension is controlled, etc. Your ongoing surveillance of each patient's medical status is paramount to a successful and healthy diet program. Follow up exams at every two weeks seem to be a safe, affordable, and acceptable time frame that has never been criticized by patients in my experience.

I think it is prudent to warn patients that an occasional patient may develop gallstones and biliary colic after significant weight loss. Any patient with such concern can be offered medication to "dissolve" gall-stones if this should occur, but there is always that patient who would never have dieted "if they had known they might get gallstones". Gouty arthritis is also an occasional result of weight loss but can be treated with medication and patients might want to know about this very infrequent complication.

Due to occasional patient problems, especially during the first 2-4 weeks, knowing the pitfalls as described in Chapter 5 on dietary supple-ments, especially with the possibility of low potassium levels from low calorie intake, can allow you to intercede and ensure that such supple-ment is being taken. Asking patients to call you during this higher risk time period usually allows the patient to resume the program and continue to make progress rather than delay it. Knowing the phenomena of patients' friends and families poor regard for your recommendation to drink "lots of diet sodas" and their countermanding it with their advice to drink "lots of water instead" leads to hyponatremia and hypokalemia and weakness. By asking if the patient has succumbed to "friendly" advice often leads to a helpful change back to your original program instructions.

Besides reading this book yourself, it is also a good idea to suggest that your patients read it as a "primer" for their weight control program. The patient will then understand that their follow up visits will not only include your medical oversight, any necessary lab tests if not feeling or doing well, and adjustments in treatment, but also discussions of patient progress in developing an alternate reward list and other behavioral modi-fication issues described throughout this book.

Although my experience is chiefly with rapid weight loss in the obese patient, and this book presents all the issues I dealt with in this subset of dieting programs, I would also recommend this book for all persons who wish to tackle a weight reduction and then weight maintenance program regardless of the amount of calorie restrictions. It remains for the physician to determine who he/she feels is qualified for a long term rapid weight reduction program. Nevertheless, in those patients with only modest caloric restrictions, this book fulfills any dieter's overall needs in succeeding with their weight control program, especially with establishing goals and behavioral modification techniques, exercise methods, and ultimately weight maintenance.

Index

One

SELF BRAINWASHING TOWARDS BETTER WEIGHT CONTROL

This diet regimen will show you how to overcome your eating impulses that have been programmed into your mind since childhood and to succeed at becoming expert, rather than average or mediocre, in your attempt to lose weight and then maintain it. The key to success should be in focusing upon far more important issues than JUST WHAT WILL I BE EATING ON THIS DIET? You probably agree that anytime someone shows interest in the latest diet, they are sure to focus simply on the food itself. What foods and how much seem to be of paramount importance in the minds of most people. In fact, the more fun or tasty the food is, the more acceptable the diet - since it would appear that losing weight and which foods to eat in accomplishing this are the prime focus. This is the fundamental (but commonplace) mistake.

In order to avoid the most common result that occurs after a weight reduction diet effort - namely, regaining all of the weight lost and following this with an insulting further weight gain - you must concentrate your efforts on certain fundamentals which modify your behavior to prevent this usual relapse. Thus, this book can help you focus on changing the innate behavior itself as the primary goal while still addressing the immediate goal of weight loss.

An analogy might be found in the following scenario. A young man states his desire to want to be a United States Marine. However, he focuses on lifting weights, running, exercise, etc. until he has developed a phenomenal muscular physique. He then cuts his hair very short, and then buys a Marine uniform from a surplus store. After presenting himself to a Marine recruiter for his "impression", it will be plainly seen that this person has been kidding himself in spite of a huge effort. The end result of his effort led only to a PHYSICAL CHANGE - not unlike the focus of most diets - eg "I want to lose 50 pounds!" However the most important component towards successfully becoming a Marine is the MENTAL CHANGE - that is, eradicating all previous civilian-acquired behavior and substituting different BEHAVIOR in its place, which transcends the physical changes in order to obtain the actually desired end-product. Obviously, this man is not even close to being a Marine!

Unfortunately, most dieters concentrate on achieving a physical change and rarely find a program which brainwashes them into achieving a new mindset regarding food itself. The usual behavior of dieters is to practice self-denial and temporarily remove food as their instant gratifier or immediate reward as long as they are happily losing weight - - - and the weight loss itself becomes their source of gratification. After sufficient weight loss occurs (or perhaps "burnout" instead), they revert back to their old ways in dealing with hunger whenever it appears, especially inappropriately.

This book will demonstrate an alternate approach which will not only lead to the immediate goal of weight loss, but far more importantly, it can lead to lasting success at weight control and attainment of personal growth. At the very beginning of my diet program with an individual patient, I tell them that their primary goal is no longer to lose X number of pounds from weight reduction alone - but to put this on the back burner of their priorities. Rather, they are told that their primary focus or purpose has henceforth changed to the following:

"I am here to learn how to become excellent at weight control during my life - and in the process

of doing this, I will also learn weight maintenance as well as the weight reduction diet. Furthermore, the above goals can be assured by automatic behavioral responses which I am about to learn. I will also learn how to become a better person during this time of hardship - - namely the weight reduction part."

The mere loss of a certain amount of weight is too superficial and insufficient for the above goals to be obtained. I have to point out that the practical result of this approach will lead to a much greater result than of just losing weight. The behavioral technique used here should ultimately broaden the spectrum of your life and enrich those moments of your lifetime that otherwise would have been enslaved to the pursuit of food. By dutifully following this approach, you will also derive a surprisingly wonderful sense of a genuinely fuller life. Dieting simply should not be a matter of temporarily withholding rewards and leaving a major void on that grand pedestal of daily gratifying rewards - only to resort back to food as the ultimate reward when the desired weight is obtained.

You will learn how to change your innate tendency to use food as your daily gratifier and to replace your pedestal of usual daily gratifiers with meaningful ALTERNATE REWARDS. The question you should ask yourself is whether or not being "skinny" is what makes you "better". Certainly, you will be healthier. But the predictable and ultimate shock and surprise of a relapse can be prevented when you actually follow this weight reduction approach which emphasizes your becoming a better person along the way. This concept should help you develop more meaning to your life and the homework involved in the behavioral modification process necessarily promotes this end. Months or years later as this part of the "diet" continues to be developed, you should be able to realize that you have become a better person - not just skinnier.

Two

Multiple Goals

There are five goals, or benefits from my approach to dieting. The first one, of course, is WEIGHT LOSS itself. This seems to be the universal goal for which everything else seems insignificant in the typical dieter. I want you to consider this as a back burner issue and not so much a major one for a change. Yet it is typical for an obese patient to get tunnel vision and focus on weight loss as his primary goal. If we focus on the other goals first, and truly concentrate on their benefits, as one proceeds on their diet, the weight will come off by default.

I listed weight loss as the first goal only because it is erroneously placed at the forefront of everyone's mind. However, secondly, but more importantly, the fundamental goal is to IMPROVE YOURSELF AS A PERSON - physically, mentally, socially, etc. Weight loss, itself, is just a superficial gift to oneself compared to the benefits of global self-improvement. It goes without saying that IMPROVING ONE'S SELF-ESTEEM is a major goal. How can this be achieved in those patients who roller-coaster their weight periodically and never prove to themselves they have got what it takes to control their weight? Following a different approach to weight control that emphasizes other goals is my answer to that dilemma.

A Physician-Patient Guidebook for a Weight Control Program

Another major goal upon which we could all could stand to improve ourselves is that of IMPULSE CONTROL. Practicing impulse control during weight reduction is certainly tedious, but becoming excellent in impulse control has benefits in all areas of our life. If, during the weight reduction experience, you focus on impulse control itself as a homework assignment for self improvement, you can see that much more than just the physical change of weight loss is accomplished. Simply stated, why not imprint into your mind how strong you are at controlling yourself when faced with major temptations and that this information builds on your self-esteem and gives you greater confidence in future situations, whether or not related to food?

Probably, the most important goal in my diet plan is that of replacing the animal-like goal for food with ALTERNATE REWARDS. Not to do this is tantamount to having a bootcamp experience - namely, changing one's behavior, undergoing rigorous physical activities, etc. and yet not lending any time towards selfish rewards. Let's face it - food is probably our most selfish and routine reward system in our life. Everyone who goes on weight reduction is denying themselves their most significant selfish reward day after day after day! In the chapter on Alternate Rewards, I will not let you get away with such a masochistic behavior. You will instead be forced to develop other personal selfish rewards - but not those which contain calories!

Lastly, your goals should be to BECOME EXCELLENT AT BOTH WEIGHT *REDUCTION* DIET methods AND WEIGHT *MAINTENANCE* DIET methods. A problem all too well experienced by repeat or burnt-out dieters is that of letting mundane problems accumulate and then in a zombie-like fashion, revert to the overeating or binge eating habits and proceed back to obesity. Utilizing what you learned in the weight reduction mode, namely, building self-esteem, impulse control, and focusing on alternate (non-caloric) rewards, which are behaviors that can take you out of your helplessness and re-institute a short-term self-imposed weight reduction mode, one can develop a sense of weight control. I will show you a method of weight maintenance that incorporates much of the weight reduction goals, but with a different emphasis on the basics. These guide-lines are far simpler than a checklist for jet aircraft take-off or landing; but if not followed, my experience is that everyone will "crash" regarding their weight control. So, making yourself a checklist of these precepts, and referring to them whenever you are falling prey to old eating behaviors are mandatory. You expect a pilot to follow such procedure - why don't you?!

Three

THE COMMONLY ACCEPTED MEANING OF DIET - WHAT FOOD - AND HOW MUCH?

Regardless of your underlying genetic predisposition towards obesity, or that you just overeat to the exclusion of other life activities, or perhaps have slowly gained too much weight as the decades have gone by, there is still only one rationale that leads to weight loss - namely eating less calories than your body uses or burns in a given time period. It is interesting how overweight people disregard this and seek out anything else that is available - from hypnotism and fad programs to exercise or aerobic schemes. This is not unlike addressing a leaky transmission in your car by spending a lot of time and trouble in changing the radiator hoses instead because they look ragged and then changing valve cover gaskets because they have a tiny leak. It would seem that such fads obviously do the dieter a favor by avoiding the key issue - FOOD RESTRICTION. However, deviating from purposeful behavior generally will not get results. Still, you see many people often succeed at weight loss while involved in any of these deviant programs - but if you add it all up, you will see that the ones who happen to lose weight are the ones that SEMI-STARVED in spite of all the other gimmicks related to their particular weight reduction scheme. The upshot to this unfortunately is that these people are programmed to fail as soon as they stop their weight reduction low calorie mode of behavior. They have learned little or nothing about how to repress their innate impulse to eat for the immediate gratification that it provides. They never learned the fundamentals of impulse-control in conjunction with the simultaneous development of non-caloric alternate rewards. Most just "gut it out" and after a suitable amount of weight has been lost, they are destined to return to FOOD as their only reward.

In fact, my approach has been the opposite of many of the so-called "cheer-leading" approaches to dieting which, for example, try to make dieting "fun" and continue to keep food on the pedestal of our daily gratifiers (ie our learned reward system). For example, the premise of "Dial a Meal" would be to insure the surprisingly-good rewards are forthcoming from tasty combinations of food albeit with the important concept of calorie restriction. Tell me where food as a major source of reward is being extinguished by this approach. There are few instant daily gratifying rewards on our immediate-rewards pedestal - but food is probably the most intensively imprinted of them all. Perhaps watching TV, socializing, games or sports, and even relieving bodily functions do serve as routine choices on that pedestal. What I am trying to do is to get you, for the first time in your life, to devalue FOOD as an important source of gratification in your daily life. While undergoing weight reduction, you should be consciously aware of such an attempt to change this behavior. In a later chapter, we will see that replacing food, as the supreme immediate-gratifier, with ALTERNATE REWARDS should serve to not only help you through the tough time of weight reduction, but that it also helps to change your tendency to automatically turn to food, especially at inappropriate times.

In my experience, starting most overweight patients on a very low calorie diet for the first week or two, regardless of their body mass index, is very therapeutic. First of all, they all demonstrate significant weight loss if they follow all instructions. Again, following exact guidelines avoids adverse side effects and the patient is rarely skeptical that further participation will lead to little progress. Unless a patient is 10 to 15 pounds or less overweight, I will usually keep them on a very low calorie diet for longer periods (and I caution them not to do vigorous exercise as long as they are on weight reduction mode). It goes without saying that patients over 40 years of age, especially high cardiovascular risk patients, diabetics, or any patient with health problems need individual attention by their physician in order to avoid a catastrophe from such physiologic stress that is placed upon them by calorie restriction. Before starting a weight reduction diet, all patients need to see their physician for a physical exam, history (including a review of systems in which to rule out any endocrine questions such as thyroid disease), and blood tests. You see, the basic considerations before starting a weight reduction diet is to determine whether or not there are reasons you should not be on such a diet. For example, you may not know that you have chronic hepatitis, anemia, chronic renal insufficiency, diabetes, high uric acid or tendency to gout, low potassium levels (especially dangerous during dieting), or other chemical abnormalities. Certain medications that you usually take could upset your body chemistry and lead to complications during an ongoing successful weight loss regimen. So, I never recommend that a patient undergo rapid or even moderate weight loss without initial medical evaluation nor without periodic followup examination and evaluation personally by a physician.

As I alluded to earlier, if you have been medically evaluated and have no contraindications to intensive weight reduction diet, I have found that a very effective approach is to start out on a very low calorie diet at least for the first week or two (or longer if you are obese.) Approximately 650 calories a day can be well tolerated if instructions are carefully followed. For two decades, I have used the following diet regimen for my weight reduction plan. If followed (without additional sources of calories that one often sneaks into the regimen) I have been satisfied with the results such that I have felt no compulsion to seek any other approach. Furthermore, it is food - not liquid protein or other unconventional diets such as powders added to skim milk, etc. Since it is easily available at the grocery store, I do not have to meddle with commercial sales of dietary weight food products. Ultimately, for a short time period of weight reduction of say, six to ten days, you can safely use this regimen on your own in the future when you need to lose a few pounds - and, you don't necessarily have to depend on some commercial or medical product source when such a short-term need arises.

650 Calorie Diet:

BREAKFAST: 1 regular glass of orange juice and 1 slice of high protein bread (such as Earthgrain's wheatberry Honey). (To avoid low blood sugar spells, divide all meals in half and take as six feedings a day instead of three - eg take the juice first thing in the morning and the bread two hours later).

ADD DIETARY FIBER to prevent "constipation". Usually patients complain of infrequent bowel movements on low calorie diets. This is simply due to less bulk ingested on such a diet. I recommend Hydrocil Instant Powder, 1 scoop mixed with the orange juice every morning. (Important to note that this powder turns to a snotty consistency after 10 seconds and therefore should be mixed in the last inch of your juice and quickly ingested).

LUNCH: Raw vegetables: cauliflower, carrots, broccoli, lettuce, cucumber, celery. After the first two weeks (remember, any lengthy low calorie regimen requires doctor followup) you may then steam the vegetables if desired. Raw vegetables, in virtually moderate amounts, are less apt to be fully digested and curtail calorie intake while still "filling" your stomach. In addition, after the first two weeks, you may add two cherry tomatoes, mushrooms, bean sprouts, bell pepper, and yellow squash. The first two weeks, you only use lemon juice or a vinegrette dressing. Thereafter, you can change to a low calorie diet dressing if not used in large amounts.

DRINKS: diet sodas

DINNER: 1 Diet TV Dinner - from 270 to 325 calories

DRINKS: diet sodas

SNACKS: Diet Sodas, LOTS (about 6/day), especially before mealtime. No caffeine preferred.

AVOID more than 2 glasses of plain water per day. DO drink 4-6 diet sodas per day. (If you are questioning this you are not alone. Read on further for the explanation. If you are being followed by a physician who is prescribing a loop diuretic such as Bumex 1mg or Lasix 40mg, you must avoid lots of plain water and take lots of diet sodas instead. Otherwise, if not on diuretics, then lots of plain water is OK.

CARRY A SMALL COOLER IN YOUR CAR WITH ICE AND DIET SODAS Also, you can keep your vegetables in plastic on ice so that you don't have an excuse for "fast food" lunches!

900 Calorie Diet:

Same as above except:

LUNCH: 1 tiny tin of chicken, turkey, or tuna (water packed) and dill pickle.

SNACKS: Add the raw vegetables listed in the 650 calorie diet at the mid-morning and mid-afternoon time slots.

There, you can see that the emphasis is not on "wonderful and tasty food" that everyone can marvel at. But it does have the potential to satisfy each individual since there is room to form-fit the food to his/her liking. Just keep in mind that **the weight *reduction* mode must emphasize the fact that you are training yourself to become a better person by taking this time to develop alternate rewards and self-esteem as well as making impulse control your conscious "homework" assignment.** If you emphasize the food over all of these primary features, then you have failed at "behavior modification."

Four

What Do You Mean by "Exercise"?

I do not recall any distinction being made, during my earlier days in training, of what exactly was meant by doing "exercise" in a diet plan. As I put markedly obese patients on a weight reduction program, I had to make the important distinction between "vigorous" and "non-vigorous" exercise in assigning patients that ever important ingredient to a weight program. What traditionally has never been taught but must be understood is that one must limit the amount of exertion a dieter performs during "weight reduction" mode as opposed to the "weight maintenance" mode.

NEVER DO VIGOROUS EXERCISE DURING WEIGHT *REDUCTION* MODE. You are depriving your body of nutrients when you curb the total calories in weight reduction mode when essentially your skeletal muscles are competing with your heart muscle (and brain) for calories. It is dangerous to run, jog, lift weights, do aerobics, or anything vigorous while you are cutting calories to lose weight in a rapid manner. Very slow weight loss programs can indeed allow some degree of vigorous exercise but my experience with rapid weight loss shows no place for this.

Therefore, one must practice "NON-VIGOROUS" EXERCISE when on weight reduction mode. What is this? Just expending more calories than usual without putting a strain on your heart and nervous system - eg standing up instead of sitting when you are on the phone, parking your car further from the entrance of your destination rather than closer, carrying in your grocery bags, etc. one at a time and making an extended effort rather than an efficient one.

I usually tell my patients during the first 2 weeks of weight reduction mode that laying around is OK because of the shock to their metabolic rate. After that, non-vigorous exercise, especially JUST WALKING, helps their weight loss in a much safer manner.

SAVE VIGOROUS EXERCISE PROGRAMS FOR WEIGHT *MAINTENANCE* MODE. Ask your doctor if it is safe since you may have been marginally safe in following a weight reduction program but adding vigorous exercise to a weight maintenance program may have to be limited.

Five

Dietary Supplements

In the preceding chapter I already alluded to the use of fiber. The most common complaint I have noted is constipation after staying on a low calorie diet. Such a change in what one ingests can surely be expected to upset your prior regularity. I have found that concentrated Psyllium fiber products prevent such complaints. Obviously, you should avoid any preparation which includes sugars, dextrose, or any calorie containing additives. I prefer Hydrocil Instant Powder - registered product- which is pure psyllium and gives the intestinal system an additional bulk to augment the lower intake you should be experiencing when on a weight reduction diet. You usually have to make a special request to your pharmacist and it will arrive the next day.

As Prenatal vitamins are important in ensuring that both the mother and growing child are not deficient in vitamins and minerals, I have prescribed them to my weight reduction patients, who are by necessity ingesting suboptimal nutrients. Such patients are just as susceptible to vitamin and mineral deficiencies as they continue on such a diet regimen. The only drawback I have seen with this is the humorous scenario of an obese cop taking his obviously marked prenatal vitamin container to the locker room with his buddies at the police station and their resultant teasing as you would imagine.

A Physician-Patient Guidebook for a Weight Control Program

The development of low blood potassium levels is especially a concern in rapid weight loss and again warrants close physician supervision. Potassium is in the form of a salt which is in all foods in varying quantities. It is normally excreted by the kidneys on a continuous basis, and this is enhanced by diuretic medications. Whether or not you eat food does not stop this excretion process. Consequently, if you are on a weight reduction diet, you are necessarily reducing your intake of potassium and there will be a point in time where your blood level of potassium becomes abnormally low unless you supplement your diet with potassium pills. Low potassium blood levels make you feel weak and sluggish and can lead to dangerous cardiac arrhythmias. Conversely, dangerous excessive accumulation of potassium blood levels, as can occur in chronic renal patients that are taking potassium supplementation, can lead to cardiac arrhythmias and death. I bring this topic up because of the need for patients, who are undergoing significant weight loss through a diet plan, to take potassium supplements AS PRESCRIBED BY THEIR DOCTOR. This avoids the weak and sluggish symptoms that will occur in a more rapid weight reduction program.

Many people feel compelled to eat bananas for their potassium supplementation - however, this is a big mistake since there are too many calories and relatively too few milliequivalents of potassium in bananas to justify using them at all. There are approximately 6 milliequivalents of potassium in one banana but unfortunately one needs about 6 bananas a day to replenish the potassium that is lacking from a low calorie diet. The calories in 6 bananas a day will cancel any benefits from a low calorie diet. Purchasing potassium pills from a health food store is not recommended since these pills are extremely low in potency and costly compared to the price of one prescription potassium pill a day that your physician can give you. One can get a false sense of security by taking 5 or 6 non-prescription potassium pills bought at a health food store, when this dose is much less than the quantity found in just one prescription potassium pill.

In my office practice, I put most of my patients on a loop diuretic while on weight reduction, require 4 to 6 diet sodas a day, and limit plain water to 2 glasses per day. It is amazing how many good intentioned "friends" of my patients tell them how wrong this is and proceed to scare them into taking lots of water and stopping the diet sodas. This can be dangerous. Let me explain, earlier I talked about normal losses of potassium from urine and the fact that a low calorie diet quite naturally deprives you of normal potassium intake. Furthermore, a diuretic causes the kidney to excrete potassium with greater intensity, regardless of how dangerously low your blood levels of potassium might be. Even more important is that blood levels of sodium are similarly excreted by the kidney and this is intensified by a diuretic. A sure way to adversely lower your sodium levels is by drinking LOTS of water AND taking a diuretic! So, following your friend's advice could lead to a seizure from low sodium levels and/or weakness and cardiac arrhythmias from low potassium levels! A physician should be sure to give you potassium supplementation by prescription while on a loop diuretic and lots of diet sodas.

Even if you are not on diuretics or diet sodas and are on a low calorie diet, after about two weeks (or sooner in many people) your blood levels of potassium drop significantly low and this in itself requires potassium supplementation. So, any healthy person that has been on a low calorie diet for an extended time, even if on no diuretics, should get potassium supplementation FROM THEIR DOCTOR in order to avoid that "washed out feeling" at the very least. However, supplemental sodium is not helpful in any regard - besides, TV dinners have sufficient if not "extra" sodium. Remember, diuretics cause sodium to be excreted. So diet sodas and TV dinners are "good" with regard to insuring adequate sodium intake and avoiding lots of water prevents dilution of both sodium and potassium levels. Everything can be in balance and thus avoid electrolyte imbalances by following your doctor's (not your friends') advice. (If you are confused, now you know why a drill instructor does not explain himself on every demand he makes - he does know that lives are saved if you do what you are told. So, if you did not understand the above, do not disregard the advice of your physician.).

A Physician-Patient Guidebook for a Weight Control Program

One must be wary of sales pitches for various and sundry products which are touted as over the counter adjuncts to weight control - especially if it has anything to do with appetite control. In the next chapter, I will explain the need for appetite-suppressant drugs, which happen to be important for the majority of obese patients and are helpful in some non-obese overweight patients. In any case, over the counter stimulants which are sold as appetite suppressants are basically decongestants (as well as caffeine products) we all are familiar with when treating a cold and are not in the same league as prescription products. To the gourmets out there, it is a little like substituting a flour tortilla in place of a crepe suzette! Just enough similarity to convince some people.

There is a recent drug, now over the counter, Alli, formerly prescriptioned as Orlistat, which does not act on the nervous system as do the appetite suppressants. It works by partially blocking the absorption of dietary fat in the gastrointestinal tract. It may play a role in the long term weight MAINTENANCE (not reduction) of patients whose metabolism mandates the use of any and all means to avoid weight gain. There are side effects such as diarrhea and smelly stools which may be too intense to tolerate. Nevertheless, this is the kind of prescription supplement to a dietary regime that could be effective once maintenance dieting begins.

If one has a normal, yet borderline elevated TSH, or Thryroid Stimulating Hormone, it might make a difference if you take a low dose of Thryoid supplement and this could assist in speeding up your metabolism rate. However, there can be harm when one takes thyroid supplement and one does **not** need thyroid supplement.

Six

APPETITE SUPPRESSION MEDICATION (OTHERWISE KNOWN AS "ANORECTICS")

Earlier I alluded to my residency training during the 1970's which claimed that anorectic drugs were "dangerous" and never to be used. After attempting to motivate obese patients to follow strict calorie restriction over an extended period of time, I came to realize that no one could achieve significant results without something to help their voracious appetites that simply would not go away under any circumstances. Since the available types of anorectics included non-amphetamine drugs such as phentermine (Fastin, Ionamin, etc.), and I was certainly against using those dangerous "amphetamines", I at least had something that was deemed less dangerous to try on these patients.

So I started using phentermine 30 mg every morning in these patients and I found they were able to tolerate the lower calorie restrictions. There were no hypertensive crises nor any mania or adverse reactions other than slightly dry mouth. The medical establishment had essentially warned us of all types of horrors - from bad cardiovascular events to "Reefer Madness" behavior, etc.- which turned out to be unfounded. If one avoids anorectics in uncontrolled hypertensives, overactive thyroid disease, or in those rare individuals that cannot tolerate them, most overweight patients in my two decades of experience can take phentermine safely and effectively. I believe the fear I had been taught that led me to avoid use of any anorectics is ungrounded specifically with the use of phentermine, which I have used almost exclusively. Interestingly, most patients do best on generic phentermine, although a few patients do better on trade-name products.

Phentermine continues to be an FDA approved weight loss medication which works by modifying the internal physiologic signals that regulate eating. More specifically, it increases brain levels of norepinephrine (which in the brain appears to decrease hunger). Contrast this drug with Dexfenfluramine (Redux) and Fenfluramine (Pondimin) which work differently by increasing serotonin levels in the hypothalamus, a part of the brain that controls the appetite. More specifically, it improves satiety. These two drugs have been taken off the market due to questions which may implicate them as a cause of heart valve problems and pulmonary hypertension. Nevertheless, my success with phentermine alone deterred my succumbing to the requests for "Phen-fen" combinations when they were in vogue during the 90's. And consequently, my patients were made to understand that the expense of such a two drug combination was unnecessary and should tolerance ever develop with phentermine alone, then perhaps it might then make sense to add another drug - to which they agreed. Wo be to those physicians that gave in to their patients who just "had to have" Phen-fen as lawyers had a hay day back then.

Controversy exists with the length of time phentermine can be prescribed. It is FDA-approved for short term use (up to three months) but there are morbidly obese patients that could never safely lose all of their excess weight in that short a time. Furthermore, it has been shown that a certain subset of obese patients essentially cannot maintain weight loss without regaining all (plus more!) their lost weight unless they take phentermine at least several days a week, if not every day. It is with these patients that the art and science of medicine come into play with their doctor's decision to extend the time that they are prescribed phentermine. There are no proven long term side effects, but extremely rare possible side effects such as primary pulmonary hypertension have led to such caution.

Dr Charles J. Neilson MD

The argument within the medical profession is the following: If the definite high risks of obesity (diabetes, cardiovascular events, hypertension, high complication risks, etc.) can be erased with a successful weight reduction and weight maintenance program, then the use of phentermine to effect this known benefit appears to outweigh any rare possibility of side effects, if they exist at all. Since the FDA has listed the use of Phentermine beyond three months as "off label", I would strongly urge physicians to write in the patient's chart that it is understood that use beyond the three months period is being carried out as long as it is still effective in bringing about weight loss. I would respect any physician that feels constrained to stop phentermine treatment after three months, but I feel any physician who would not ever use phentermine in obese patients is still living in the 1970's. You can find a physician that does use phentermine, but do not be surprised if he/she stops your prescription if you waste your opportunity to curb your appetite in an efficient manner.

Concerning anorectics as a "tool" to assist you in losing weight, one must realize that the job can not be successful if total reliance is on the "tool" itself. You must concentrate on developing alternate rewards that lead to enhanced self esteem and personal growth. This is why every patient that goes to a doctor and gets an appetite-suppressant, loses weight, and then regains it back, plus more, is not only wasting his time, but increasing the likelihood of decreasing his self-esteem. You simply can not rely on anorectics alone to achieve your weight loss goals, because such a superficial approach is a guarantee to fail - and quite understandably, you will develop a mental picture of yourself as a failure at weight control. Yes, you may be a successful businessperson, well-liked, talented, etc. but as long as you insist on tackling your weight control problem in a simplistic one-dimensional approach ("pills"), each failure is a reminder that reinforces your self-portrait as unquestionably destined to always be obese. But on the other hand, using "pills" to suppress appetite is a bit like using an electric saw in carpentry so as to make a hard job somewhat easier.

Another anorectic which has FDA-approved indications for both weight reduction and maintenance of weight loss is Sibutramine (Meridia).

It increases both serotonin and norepinephrine levels by inhibiting their reuptake by nerve cells. Dexfenfluramine and Fenfluramine increases serotonin in a different manner by increasing the release of serotonin only. Phentermine increases the release of norepinephrine. To date there is no evidence of adverse heart valve problems or other serious considerations and my intention is to use Sibutramine as a long term weight maintenance drug treatment for formerly obese patients who feel that this FDA-approved indication makes it more favorable or technically less risky than Phentermine.

Another drug similar to phentermine is Phendimetrazine (Bontril) which comes in regular and slow-release doses. Due to some variances in patient responses, I will occasionally use this instead of phentermine. A common problem of tolerance develops with these drugs and after several weeks a patient may not get as good appetite suppression as he/she did initially, and slow-release forms can be tried or an additional 15 milligrams of phentermine can be given around 3:30 pm (Ionamin 15 mg.) with good results.

Seven

Development of Impulse Control

Remember that there are a number of "fundamental" behaviors or goals with which to develop while you are on a weight reduction program. Your overall goal is to achieve excellence in these behavioral or thought patterns besides just losing weight. I do not have to argue how important it is for you to become excellent at impulse control if you are interested in becoming excellent at weight control lifelong. Since "practice makes perfect", you will have to look at all of those expected temptations and challenging situations as "homework exercises" for development of impulse control rather than obstacles that stand in your way.

What is the requirement for obtaining excellence in any human endeavor? Certainly hard work is part of the equation. Never discount the importance of a great challenge. Suppose you wanted to be excellent in tennis. You would not choose a fairly good player as your mentor/instructor over the likes of a big-name tennis star if you had the chance, would you? Sometimes we have to force ourselves to appreciate the benefits of taking on a great challenge. For example, if you were in high school and you wanted to be a math major in college as well as a cheerleader or some other time-consuming activity during your senior year, and you had a choice between Mrs Grundy, the hardest math teacher, and Ms. Smythe,

the easiest math teacher, who would you pick? It is obvious that the greater obsessive-compulsive learning experience from Mrs Grundy would have prepared you for the competition in college you are certain to see from those students who had greater challenges in high school. This line of thinking presupposes your quest to be excellent in math. If this is not your goal, then such choices may be different. But my diet approach presupposes that you are seeking to develop excellence in weight control!

In obese patients, any attitude short of desiring to become excellent in the fundamentals of weight control will lead to mediocrity - which in many patients means failure. Not acquiring a track record of excellence in impulse control hurts you far worse than just from the immediate consequences that occur by prolonging the weight reduction phase. For example, if your memory bank is imprinted with intermittent half-hearted episodes of meeting the temptations of daily food choices, especially during the weight reduction phase of dieting, then you have very little positive information with which to recall at a later date when you must rely on your stored memories of excellence at impulse control. Imagine trying to avoid uncontrolled eating during next years' Christmas holiday season and having imprinted in your brain a less than optimal impulse control experience during the weight reduction phase (where fundamentals are to be learned and practiced well.) Let's face it, if you cheated a lot during the inception of this diet program, then your ability to recall behavioral excellence (along with the inner rewarding consequences) will be deficient when major temptations enter into your life. Conversely, if you were able to develop a successful series of excellent impulse control experiences in your memory bank, then future temptations could be more easily sidestepped. Furthermore, I know of no one whoever felt bad about themselves when they walked away from food temptations successfully.

Now, all of this impulse control homework is to be practiced during the weight reduction mode. I'll give you an example: Suppose you have lost 20 pounds and you are not yet near your ideal weight, but closing in on it. Your spouse just received a $300 coupon for both of you towards a fine evening at your town's finest gourmet restaurant but only for tonight.

No rainchecks! If you are "normal" you would rationalize that "this is only one meal" and that it could not make that great a dent in your progress, that you could never afford such an opportunity without the coupon, etc. etc. etc. My approach to behavioral modification is to emphasize that you are essentially in "boot camp" at this time and you are learning the fundamentals with which to fight the "war" (ie your weight)and that reverting back to old behaviors and thinking patterns during this critical point in "training" disrupts the finished product. Making this scenario an exercise in which to develop impulse control excellence instead of a repeat performance of "giving in" to temptation is crucial toward your own personal "brainwashing". Regardless, whether or not you send your sister in your place, or make a pact with your spouse to acknowledge your intention to just eat a salad, fish, and bottled water ONLY, this will have been a wonderful opportunity to practice impulse control. After succeeding at this, you will be evermore certain of your newfound excellence in impulse control. Just who out there in the world could do what you just did?! Months or years later, when you feel trapped by overwhelming temptation, all you have to do is remind yourself of how strong you were in not falling prey to this temptation of all temptations.

The major point I am trying to make is that when you undertake a weight reduction diet, there are other goals in which to achieve excellence besides fast or smooth weight loss - and one of the most important is to acquire excellence in impulse control. To succeed with the former (weight loss), you have to succeed in the latter (impulse control). However, there is more to think about regarding just succeeding at calorie restriction by holding back and "white knuckling" every temptation that arises. You have to appreciate those horrendous inhuman scenarios which require you to exhibit extra strength in self-denial as being just homework exercises necessary to prime your memory bank with positive experiences that will make future temptations easier to withstand. And when such a great challenging temptation makes itself present, you can look at it forthrightly and say "Great! This is what I need to develop excellence in impulse control." It's your recollection of successfully withstanding the strongest temptations that you are really able to improve your willpower and forever remind yourself of excellence in impulse control.

There are certain scenarios that invariably lead to failure if you are not forewarned. I have seen many an obese female make excellent progress in weight reduction or maintenance only to have her obese relatives or obese colleagues at work, etc. sabotage her effort by tempting her incessantly. I believe a certain psychological dynamic causes this common-place problem. The mere fact that my patient is succeeding at such a difficult task is disconcerting to these people and being human (competitive? jealous? etc.) they assume my patient wrongfully has the opinion that she is better than them and actually is succeeding at what they themselves have not been able to accomplish. They know my patient is going through a charade and that ultimately she will find out, as they have, that she too is "weak" and will come down to reality. How dare she demonstrate that she has great character and impulse control and the like. "Well, I'll show her she is no better than myself.!" As a result we see an onslaught of sweets, pastries, free take-out lunches from co-workers, and snooty reactions if this is un-welcomed. With this line of thinking, you can only maintain your friendships if you relent and start regaining weight again. This will ease their mind and reassure them that weight loss/control is impossible and thereby relieve them of the very thought of having to go on a diet themselves. Such a quest in which to test their own character is definitely not on their agenda. But my patients have been counseled to recognize these pitfalls and they are not only responsible to themselves but as leaders to their unhappy obese friends. The key responsibility is in conveying to them that denying themselves the personal everyday selfish reward system comprised of just food and replacement of this with alternate rewards (next chapter) and practicing impulse control and boosting self-esteem outweigh the negative experiences of denying oneself unlimited food rewards.

Now, what about the Thanksgiving scenario where you find yourself facing a cornucopia of wonderful food set on the table by mom, who has spent hours in the kitchen preparing all of this? Why do you suppose mom tells you to "Get out of the kitchen" while she slaves away all morning long? Could it be that in our culture, this is an indirect way of telling our loved-ones how much she loves them - with the toil of preparation being the proof. And when you sit down finally and view the culmination of all this loving toil, imagine the reaction of not only mom, but the whole family, when you retort that you are on a diet and cannot dare eat much of anything! This is a slap in the face and in an uncouth way fails to reciprocate the love that has emanated from our dear mom. Anybody in his right mind would, out of such guilt, pour on their plate seconds and thirds, as it were, rather than feel the recriminations from carrying out a more limited intake. Why?

Because we do not understand that we can still reciprocate our love back to mom and the family in other formats besides chowing down, making gustatory noises of appreciation, and grabbing more and more food to communicate our love, you can still reciprocate your love in a verbal manner without overdoing the feeding routine. You can bring to the table loving thoughts and thanks to everyone and even bring thoughtful gifts or old family pictures, etc. Your goal when asked why you aren't stuffing yourself is not to say you are on a diet, but to overwhelm everyone with verbal communications of love. That is really what Thanksgiving, Christmas, Birthday, and any other holiday family dinner is all about.

A word about business lunches and dinners, banquets, etc. is important. These may not be social rituals in which to express love, but they nevertheless appear to be reward systems meant for employees and customers. Again, to deny yourself a full-fledged restaurant meal at no cost to yourself is somewhat of a slap in the face to the host or client. Your quest is again to reciprocate good will and try to avoid the consumption of food as the predominant method of effecting this. Charming verbal communication and thoughtful pleasantries can and should prove that your failure to fill up your plate is not symbolic of some discomfiture.

Eight

DEVELOPMENT OF SELF ESTEEM

Rather than actual weight loss, it is paramount that you focus on a number of goals to be achieved while going through the process of cutting calories, taking appetite suppressants, potassium supplements, and whatever else is part of the actual weight reduction protocol. One of the goals that should be constantly remembered is that during all of this hardship, there are many opportunities to develop positive self-esteem. Not only are we trying to develop self-esteem from achievement and/or development of alternate rewards (to be discussed in a later chapter) but as a specific goal, we should derive greater self-esteem from the knowledge that successfully following the guidelines of weight reduction and weight maintenance is in itself an important goal. Why is this?

One of the most common obstacles that prevents starting up or maintaining a diet program for obese people is their incessant negative self-image. Each successive dietary failure in their personal history is stored in their gray matter "memory bank" and in spite of their other wonderful achievements, they can always compute from their diet data experiences that they are programmed to fail whenever they undertake a diet program. You can blame your obesity on genetics, God, or whatever, but the facts are that in spite of how great you may be in all other aspects of your being, you feel that you are a loser when it comes to long term weight control.

Therefore it is imperative that when undertaking this current weight program, that you be clear-minded that not only is excellence in closely following the diet program important to get the weight off, but more importantly, this is the time in which you imprint into your memory bank the fact that you are excellent at weight reduction itself. Everyone knows the unlikelihood of a high school dropout to eventually get a college diploma. What chance is there when an average intellect has stored in his mind nothing but negative academic experiences. The key is in turning around from a series of failing behavior to excellent behavior. So, once you take on the diet program this time, **you must concentrate on the fact that this an experience where there is no room for fooling around - and that it is a serious matter in which you are actually undergoing a psychological exercise to imprint a series of positive data within your memory bank in which to retrieve for the future.** Imagine succeeding in an excellent manner this time and then finding yourself in a depressed state of mind a year later but able to remember that you can truly feel great (instead of more depressed) just by forcing yourself to "do the right thing" - and that having confidence in yourself can only give you such impetus to succeed. It is commonplace for those obese patients that roller coaster their weight up and down to resign themselves to failure just because they never experienced a succession of excellent weight control behavior over a reasonable period of time. One must imprint into their brain the fact that they ARE excellent at weight control. I am reminded of what one short boot camp experience can do to all of those young Marine recruits. If there is one thing many of them have experienced for the first time in their life, it is self-esteem, self-confidence, and a strong desire not to fail. My recollection of why this happens is that drill instructors never accept deficiencies or negative characteristics and that each individual has to focus on overcoming whatever his personal deficiency may be. No excuses! It is a rare recruit who does not have a number of spiritual awakenings regarding how great it feels to be able to do whatever he lacked confidence in himself to be able to do in the past. Look at how long such a behavioral system lasts when we think of the saying "once a Marine, always a Marine".

A byproduct of this experience has worked well for my patients over the years after they learned my weight control system. Namely, in those individuals who are prone to depression and then automatically seek food as a learned response, I have impressed upon them how reinforcement of their positive self-image and reinstitution of their prior excellent impulse-control behavior actually works as anti-depressant therapy. And this costs no money, is not in a pill, and starts working almost immediately rather than two weeks later (as seen from anti-depressant pills.) The upshot is that you must have a baseline positive experience of excellence which includes following orders, so to speak. If you think you are different or so special as to merit deviation from a system that works well, then your self-confidence when needed down the road will be lacking. This is human nature. If I told you that I failed anatomy in medical school, you probably would lose confidence in me as a physician. But more importantly, how would I feel about myself as a physician if it were true? The truth is that I made "Best Student in Anatomy". So, now you feel some relief from that fact, but more importantly my self-esteem is certainly reassured.

So, what if you have all kinds of genetic and cultural disadvantages that make your weight problem truly a greater obstacle to overcome than is found in most people? The answer lies in the phenomenon called "overcompensation". You are not the only ones in this world that have to overcompensate to achieve excellence in a desired area. Take those small-statured or small-framed recruits who seem to do quite well as compared to the occasional muscular, handsome picture-perfect Marine recruit that never gave 100% effort in his life and during bootcamp is unwilling to carry his load and fails (and has to live with this failure for the rest of his life.) Look at stutterers who become famous singers or top notch network commentators. ***All the obese patient needs to concentrate on is the fact that performing in an excellent manner, without demonstrating weakness, is the first step toward imprinting positive information with***

which to retrieve in future tough situations. Think about the incessant car thief who just gets out of prison and then goes out and steals your car. Imagine how mad you would be as well as how depressed and chagrined the thief would be after being caught once again and being re-incarcerated. I would imagine that if asked why he made the same errant behavior again, he would say "I guess that's just the way I am - I can't change that part of me." Naturally, you would expect that several jail sentences should make him change his behavior for the better. But it doesn't! And we are incensed at this illogical and stupid behavior. Then when we personally continue to spiral down and down the path of failure time and time again and imprinting nothing but negative self-image (but limited to our weight control capabilities), we are behaving the same way as that car thief whom we despise. No wonder obese people, that have never succeeded at weight control, are sensitive to outside pressure that implies that they are failures. Again, there are wonderful and positive physical changes which do indeed occur to recruits in boot camp, but these changes occur in conjunction with major changes in behavior and self-image.

Earlier, I stated that any diet program which cuts calories will lead to weight reduction. The most important issue is that this weight loss will be short-lived if the diet regimen does not, like the boot camp experience, include behavioral modification and enhanced self-esteem. In chapter nine I will point out the greatest way to enhance self-esteem and impulse control, namely by developing a list of alternate rewards (in place of food).

Nine

ALTERNATE REWARDS

As I have mentioned throughout this book, to lose weight without replacing the loss of pleasure one gets from the un-curtailed ingestion of delicious food is a major mistake. Since food appears to be the primal immediate gratifier in our basic reward system, most dieters do indeed set out to punish themselves by denying themselves food for as long as their willpower permits. Never, but never, do they conceptualize that by removing this dominant immediate gratifier, they really MUST seek out alternate rewards. Furthermore, these alternate rewards must be non-caloric in nature. When in boot camp, you suffer privations of the most basic sort, such as not being able to eat when and what you desire, not going to the rest room ad lib, no watching television, no reading, socializing, etc. I'll just bet that the main reason most young people avoid military training and service is not because of some danger in defending the country, but because of simply being denied those basic immediate gratifiers, especially during the temporary boot camp experience.

It is obvious that those who contemplate dieting similarly cannot bear to give up their basic primal needs. Could it be that what the dieter needs that the bootcamp experience cannot offer is the opportunity, no REQUIREMENT, that during this diet regime, they be forced to seek alternate rewards? There is no need to suffer such deprivation when one consciously replaces the loss of food as one's immediate gratifier with a growing list of alternate rewards which ultimately lead one toward overall personal development. The consolation prize in this approach is that, oh yes, you lose weight, look better, live healthier and longer, etc. But during the weight reduction phase, you began a process of self-growth that opens the door to an even better life. After all, being skinny in and of itself, does not make you a better person except in a constrained manner of speaking. Go for it all! My approach to dieting requires you to consciously develop a multitude of interesting activities, hobbies, intellectual pursuits, avocations, and areas of expertise which build on your self-esteem as well as to succeed in quick and sustained weight loss. There are many people in our current society that have been processed through a "new wave" educational process which does not foster a competitive spirit of excellence and achievement. This is unfortunate since it would appear that self-esteem is only derived from some nebulous mental conceptualizations as well as not being fat.

I often ask individuals with weight problems as well as other personal problems, such as marital or relationship problems, what is or are the things that they are excellent at doing. Quite often there is an astounding lack of pursuit in any areas of life's activities. Even those people who do socialize vigorously often do not claim any one area of expertise or even a quest to develop self-respect and command the respect of others by having made the effort towards excellence per se. I can see a group of adolescents "hanging out" at the Mall and the kind of reaction one of those kids might receive from the rest of the group if he/she stated "I'll see you all tomorrow, I've got to go to my flamenco guitar lessons". Well, imagine the repartee - such as "Who do you think you are? Some kind of Spaniard or something?" With such peer pressure to hang out with the gang in high school and essentially being made to feel a lack of self-esteem when seeking personal growth and evoking the wrath of one's peers, it's no wonder there is no zeal for self-growth in our society. Likewise, I have found that many dieters lack any understanding of what is expected of them when they are "ordered" to seek out alternate rewards as a major exercise in the weight reduction regimen. It is interesting that they will only write on their list such things as "shopping" or "reading a novel." Although such things conceivably might be a true alternate reward, there is a hint of lack of desire to really grow as a person and experience life to the fullest that God gives one the talent to pursue.

There is one adjective that must be considered when developing a list of Alternative Rewards and this is the word "SELFISH". Just as food is a selfish immediate gratifier for each of us, likewise, you should seek out selfish alternate rewards on your list as a means to effectively replace that exponent of selfishness which you are denying yourself while on a diet. You may like sauerkraut and string beans on your hamburger and I could care less - but it is YOUR selfish gratifier nevertheless. Many times I have had patients followup with me after two weeks and not have anything written on their Alternate Reward List. When asked why, they have even tearfully confessed that there was absolutely NOTHING that they could think of that they wanted to develop as a replacement reward for food. There you have it, they are willing to gut it out, deprive themselves of their only real reward, FOOD, and as soon as some weight is lost, resume personal gratification from delicious food and regain all their lost weight. This is when I help them understand that they cannot blame their obesity on a multitude of unfair hardships, genetics, etc. - but that the major obstacle is that NOTHING in their life is as important or rewarding as is FOOD! At this point we can work towards success when we assist each individual in developing selfish personal non-caloric rewards.

Occasionally, a psychiatrist has to be consulted in order to help those with a mental block against self-growth. The sine qui none of successful long term diet regimes in my experience, and in my patients' opinions, is that conscious development of selfish alternate rewards.

The following is a copy of my handout which I give out the first visit on my weight program. You might be surprised that most people do not write it down on paper as I repeatedly tell them to do and even state on this handout! As in bootcamp, when you do not do as you are told (when you are essentially being brainwashed) you miss out on the full benefits of the program. In war, you get yourself killed if you do not heed your drill instructor's command with implicit faith. For the obese patient, the war is with their weight, and there is little chance for success when the "recruit" thinks he is so special as to warrant special privileges in maneuvering through the diet regime to suit their individual personal needs. In my first two decades of medical professional experience regarding dieting, this analogy is absolutely operative. Therefore, if you find extreme difficulty in just listing a number of alternative rewards over several weeks, then you will ultimately find that food is your only significant selfish reward in life and in spite of a temporary loss of weight, you are destined to resume uncontrolled eating habits as you rightfully seek the reinstitution of rewards you have so painstakingly omitted from your life while dieting.

ALTERNATE REWARD LIST - A MORE FULFILLING MENU FOR YOUR LIFE:

I always ask why people feel compelled to look at the menu when at a restaurant, especially one that they really like and yet already know what they want. However, if I were to tell you that you could not read the menu at a seafood restaurant (where you always order fried shrimp) while the rest of us at the table read ours, you would be upset. How unfair! It is almost as if having that menu, even with knowing what you want, is an important part of the behavioral process of enjoying a pleasurable meal. It is this very important item we refer to in the process of starting off our gustatory glee that I want you to emphasize. The MENU. Well, an Alternate Reward List is in essence a MENU for a happy life - and a necessity in weight control behavior. If you do not have an Alternate Reward List to refer to when you are craving food or about to fall prey to temptation to eat unnecessarily, then you are depriving yourself of a guide that will help you redirect your requisite need

for selfish rewards that you receive from food. You **MUST** have an ongoing and growing **ALTERNATE REWARD LIST** on your person in which to refer to during any episode of relentless hunger or desire to "get off the wagon". This list of alternative rewarding activities should remind you of many things to do that are selfishly pleasurable but are **NON-CALORIC** in nature. Such rewarding activities should include old or new hobbies, learning to play or developing a musical instrument capability, singing, or whatever talent you possess that gives you a sense of self-esteem as you become more accomplished. Writing poetry, etc., bowling, becoming a self-styled "expert" in some area of interest you hold, or **WHATEVER** deep hidden God-given talent or interest you possess. The key here is that it is **YOUR** interest that must be developed. Just as Elvis gorged lustfully on peanut butter and fried banana sandwiches, who am I to tell him what far out food should give him pleasure? Likewise, who am I to tell you what to put on your **ALTERNATE REWARD LIST**. As described above, there are people who simply **CANNOT** make such a list. They have unrequited talents, but have allowed food, social life, shopping, television, internet, and likely sex to provide the basis for rewards in their behavioral system. I tell them after the first 2 weeks that they **MUST** start writing a few items down on their menu that they feel will make their life more pleasurable or rewarding and ultimately would lead to further interest to the point of developing extreme excellence. As they think of things they used to like, to things they currently like, to things they never knew they would like - and by process of selection eventually develop a sense of reward and self-esteem from this development of a broader life. What better than leaving a legacy such as "grandma was the expert in the county on.." this or that or "she was like Grandma Moses, ..." she did not start painting until she was in her 50's".

Unfortunately, many a patient returns after four weeks on the diet WITHOUT starting a list of items, even after my first "warning". Not even one item! They often cry and feel inadequate, if not hopeless, with regard to this quest that I make very clear to them. This is when I remark, "You should know that the reason you are obese and unable to control your weight is not because of hormones, genes, family background, or anything out of your control, but because YOU CANNOT find anything else, besides food, from which to derive pleasure. You will simply have to force yourself to develop other sources of pleasure and self-esteem in order to succeed." Whether the result of social pressure or culturally learned behavior, many people sacrifice their self growth by not ever developing selfish rewarding activities. Some people think they must coordinate their hobby or selfish interest with their spouse or do nothing at all. Family pressure often suppresses ventures into self development to the point of being made to feel like a selfish spouse. Yet, a wife's mother-in-law does not mind if the wife eats to the point of obesity as long as she is a domestic slave to her family. Such pressure to derive pleasure from eating as the sole reward source is rampant and must be overcome.

Get this straight: If you cannot slowly develop personal and selfish rewarding activities, and write them down, and cross some out after finding out their lack of pleasure, and add to the list, to make a dynamic menu that you can refer to whenever you need to offer yourself an immediate (or delayed) gratifier, then you will have learned nothing during the weight reduction mode and then fall prey to food as the only source of gratification when weight maintenance comes around. On the other hand, with your ongoing and growing "menu for life", you will have developed a list of items, some of which embellish your life and provide growing self-esteem- thus becoming a BETTER PERSON. Losing weight alone does not make you a better person. Using my behavior approach should help you actually become a better person by opening up self growth and talents while you are losing weight and learning to control it.

Ten

Weight Maintenance

After you have completed your weight reduction diet mode, or even more importantly, when you decide to temporarily stop the weight reduction diet, you must follow a somewhat different diet modality - namely weight maintenance. This does entail an increase in calories, though not a free for all, unbridled return to old undisciplined dietary habits. This is a specific regimen which mandates a continued mental process as practiced in the weight reduction mode - namely, development of alternate rewards. Other adjustments must be made when greater calorie intake occurs. For example, the type of exercise in weight maintenance should change to vigorous rather than non-vigorous. This would be the time to join a health club or buy health equipment, swim laps, jog, etc. The initiation of such vigorous activity needs to be authorized by your personal physician as alluded to in chapter four.

You should note that I never advocate daily weight checks during weight reduction because at this time I am trying to condition you to extinguish the innate tendency for weight loss itself as being your primary goal towards replacing it with the development of an alternate rewards system instead. Knowing what you weigh on a daily basis is as important to the whole process as measuring your bicep and neck muscles on a daily basis in boot camp. I can assure you that in both cases you will be amply satisfied at the end of the process if you simply concentrate on the discipline of just following orders. How much you lose from day to day is not important - rather how much you lose over two week increments is what matters. Besides, if you follow your calorie intake exactly, develop an alternate rewards list, exercise, and notify your physician of any problems that might tend to make you alter the diet, then you are going to most likely lose more weight than you ever have in the past.

However, **DAILY WEIGHING during weight MAINTENANCE IS REQUIRED** so as to avoid significant weight-gain surprises. You must reject the commonplace behavior of refusing to weigh yourself for many weeks out of fear of knowing just how much weight you have gained. The longer you wait, guarantees depression and possibly another tedious uphill battle. Just simply weigh and follow your written check list and then you can rest assured that you are "in control" rather being controlled.

It is obvious that you should eat more calories on weight maintenance than weight reduction. How much more you should be eating during weight maintenance can be gauged by any noticeable weight gain over several days. As seen in my handout for weight maintenance, I indicate the **"66 Rule"** which mandates resumption of the low calorie weight reduction diet for 6 days IF you have gained 6 pounds from your baseline level. If you keep a close eye on your daily weight, you can avoid the rule of 66 by cutting back on your intake just one meal if needed. Furthermore, the baseline weight will probably have to be increased by 5-8 pounds depending on how much muscle weight is gained during the vigorous exercise experienced during weight maintenance. Such weight gain is healthy and occurs in areas that do not involve the waistline. This is a natural phenomenon and makes up for muscle wasting that occurs from rapid weight loss.

What kind of food is best for weight maintenance? A general rule would be high protein, low fat and moderate carbohydrates. Just how much starch or carbohydrates should be finely tuned by the degree of vigorous exercise versus any weight gain that develops. This should vary according to each person's metabolic rate. It can be simply said that after a person has been on weight reduction (low calories) for a while, his metabolism (or calorie burning efficiency) "slows down." **This means that resumption of what was his previous "normal" maintenance intake (ie prior to dieting) becomes excessive in the face of this newly acquired metabolic slowdown.** Consequently, people that struggle to lose weight successfully invariably blame themselves for regaining all of their lost weight (plus more) when their maintenance calorie intake does not seem to be anymore than what used to suffice for maintenance before they started weight reduction! But the vigorous exercise and the slow and careful increase in calories during weight maintenance is important while waiting for the metabolic rate to speed up.

In spite of breads being one of the basic food groups, I am never surprised by the need for patients with weight problems to overeat breads, citing the so-called importance of satisfying this food group requirement. I have to say that some people may have to over-compensate for their genetic proclivity to gain weight by "just saying no" to breads in general. For example, eating no garlic toast with spaghetti, removing one of the buns on their hamburger, eating sandwiches with thin high protein bread only, etc.

Another part of weight maintenance that most people will fail to do unless it is emphasized, is to continue to develop and practice their alternate reward list. Also, failure to see their doctor every three months can deter continuing success. Invariably, when I see someone who failed to come in for followup, after, say eight to twelve months, they have regained some weight, gotten frightened, and in every case, forgot about their alternate reward goals, stopped exercising, and fell into old habits without even following the systematic changes they once mastered. This certainly illustrates the the power of food as the number one selfish gratifier and how it can mesmerize you into failure. Furthermore, by seeing your physician every three months, he may provide you with a prescription for several phentermine capsules to be used at strategic moments when weight reduction should be carried out. Weintraub's studies even pointed out that the unfortunate marked obese patients will in fact gain back a considerable amount of weight if they do not take an appetite suppressant medication routinely. I have personally found that this amount varies from one person to the next, with some requiring three pills a week, especially on weekends, and others four pills a week, especially during the work week. Some just need a few pills sporadically. The previously non-obese with milder weight problems do not need routine anorectic treatment. I have already spoken earlier about the fact that long term use of anorectic medication (as used in weight maintenance for the previously marked obese patients) is done so with the patient being informed that there are no known significant side effects with the long term use of phentermine yet, on the other hand, there are considerable risks if obesity recurs - eg. hypertension, diabetes, cardiac disease, greater complication rates after surgery, etc. So, finding a physician that appreciates this need for markedly obese patients to take phentermine on a long term regimented basis may be the only way (along with exercise, alternate reward behavior, and the other behavior patterns, such as the "rule of 66") for these individuals to keep from regaining alot of weight. There is no place for the average patient to rely on such anorectic medications on a regular basis.

If you find that your weight has creeped up six pounds, then you must follow the weight reduction strict calorie diet mode for six days. However, by checking your weight EVERY DAY during weight maintenance, you may notice a pattern of weight gain (eg. only three or four pounds) and can elect a more ad lib form of calorie restriction. In either case, such a situation MUST call forth for a reflexive contemplation of the Alternate Reward List behavior pattern. You have been truly "brain washed" like the military if you have made a conscious effort during weight reduction to instill this behavior. It should be as automatic as a Marine saluting an officer when he walks by at any time. It is interesting that there is punishment for disobeying this basic rule in the military yet with a formerly obese civilian patient who stands to be "punished" by regaining considerable weight by not remembering to follow the Alternate Rewards behavior one must consider the fact that here the "punishment" is not swift in coming.

So, one must develop a conscious reflexive behavior that automatically recalls the exact mental state that led to previous success. You should be an optimist when this happens and tell yourself that the difference between forcing yourself back into a "bootcamp" self-denial experience as opposed to the weight reduction mode of thinking is that you have been conditioned to behave in a way that fosters multiple sources for self-gratification. On the contrary, there is no place for alternate reward self-gratification in bootcamp or the brig, for that matter. Why should you feel punished from self-imposed denial of great tasting food IF you have made a conscious effort to practice the alternate reward concept more closely for the next few days? Again, I allude to the analogy of the pilot's checklist for landing a 747. There is no room for disregarding this systematic approach when considering the dangers of a crash. So, for those patients have a history of "crashing" every time they successfully lose weight, I recommend that they carry a copy of my office handout for Weight Maintenance and follow it when there is the slightest notion of "Oh boy! Here I go again!"

For those selected patients with difficulty in maintaining their weight, I feel that the use of Orlistat to lower the amount of fat that is absorbed from their maintenance diet can be useful. You may have to ask your physician to prescribe this however, plus you might suffer from fatty stools, diarrhea, etc.- all reasons why I do not recommend this during weight reduction phase. Nevertheless, anything to help prevent your weight from creeping up after your successful reduction effort is worth a try. Earlier I mentioned in chapter six the possibility of using Sibutramine (Meridia) for appetite suppression in the maintenance phase although I personally have not used it at all. It may carry approval for long term maintenance in States where phentermine is not allowed for maintenance use.

Final Considerations

This book is the result of my experience as a family physician and, in particular, as a medical practitioner who successfully helped hundreds of patients with a weight problem. Since most of my weight program was developed on my own and was not part of my formal training, I can attest that the foregoing nevertheless worked better than I had ever hoped for. Unfortunately, todays practitioners' training, like mine, may still not include all of the particulars that are needed to guide their patients along in a weight program. So, I am hoping that your knowledge of these necessary components will help you and your physician make your weight control program a success. As I have said before, you cannot perform this on your own and must have a doctor prescribing medicines like Phentermine, potassium supplements, vitamins, and the actual food/calories, as well as a behavior modification program, along with the appropriate exercise modality. After reading this book, you should be able to see your family physician or primary care doctor for an even better experience in weight control.

My personal peeve is any specialty weight program that continues to keep food on the pedestal to worship and keep as the highest reward system without ever replacing it with non-caloric alternatives. On the contrary, my approach actually worked fabulously in my practice and with your doctor's help, you can be an "expert" at weight control. **By expert, I mean that *you not only know how to do weight reduction and weight***

maintenance in an excellent manner, but that the process requires you to better yourself personally, so that you do not just lose weight. Being skinnier is not being better.........unless you develop personal alternative rewards, impulse control, self esteem, and improve yourself as a person. Everything required to meet that goal was included in my program. You and your physician have a relationship that does not preclude your input toward attaining your medical goals. As far as weight control, you now have covered the comprehensive experience of one family physician that had enormous positive experiences for two decades with all his weight patients.

About the Author

Charles J. Neilson MD, FAAFP is a native 6th Generation Texan, former Marine, and Vietnam Veteran who graduated from UCLA and obtained his medical degree from the Albany Medical College of Union University in upstate New York. He came back home to Texas to attend Baylor College of Medicine in Houston where he studied Family Medicine. He has continued his association with the American Academy of Family Physicians as a Fellow of the AAFP. He was a preceptor to 116 medical students in his office practice after he began a traditional solo private family practice in Houston in 1977. After 21 years he changed to full time emergency medicine which he has practiced since 1999. His experience as an emergency physician has included being a pioneer as the Medical Director of the only real time 24 hour a day rural hospital emergency telemedicine operation in Texas (one of three nationally) in 1999-2004. His development of an effective and safe rapid weight loss program began when he was serving the Houston Police Department as their Boxing Team physician and several overweight policemen asked him for professional help to lose weight. He found out that what he had just learned in residency did not work and he quickly reformulated a program that did work. The satisfied patients' word of mouth helped his program grow until it became a big part of his practice. He has lived in Sugar Land, Texas, a suburb of Houston, since 1985. He has been married for 36 years and has three grown children.